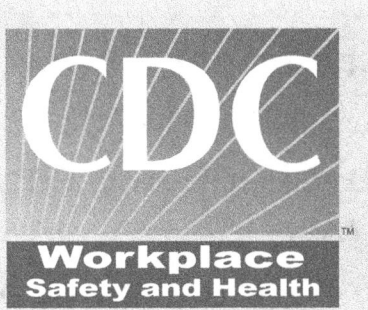

I0415796

Evaluation of Police Officers' Exposures to Chemicals While Working Inside a Drug Vault – Kentucky

Kenneth W. Fent, PhD
Srinivas Durgam, MSPh, MSChE, CIH
Christine West, RN, MSN, MPH
John Gibbins, DVM, MPH
Jerome Smith, PhD

Health Hazard Evaluation Report
HETA 2010-0017-3133
July 2011

DEPARTMENT OF HEALTH AND HUMAN SERVICES
Centers for Disease Control and Prevention

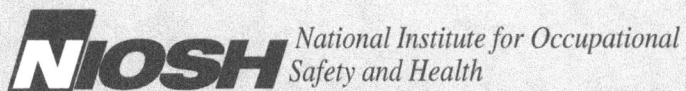

National Institute for Occupational
Safety and Health

The employer shall post a copy of this report for a period of 30 calendar days at or near the workplace(s) of affected employees. The employer shall take steps to insure that the posted determinations are not altered, defaced, or covered by other material during such period. [37 FR 23640, November 7, 1972, as amended at 45 FR 2653, January 14, 1980].

CONTENTS

ABBREVIATIONS

ACGIH®	American Conference of Governmental Industrial Hygienists
AIHA	American Industrial Hygiene Association
ANSI	American National Standards Institute
ASHRAE	American Society of Heating, Refrigerating, and Air-Conditioning Engineers
C	Ceiling limit
cfm	Cubic feet per minute
cfm/ft²	Cubic feet per minute per square foot
CFR	Code of Federal Regulations
°F	Degrees Fahrenheit
ft²	Square foot
HEPA	High efficiency particulate air
HHE	Health hazard evaluation
HVAC	Heating, ventilating, and air-conditioning
MDC	Minimum detectable concentration
mg/m³	Milligrams per cubic meter
mm	Millimeter
MQC	Minimum quantifiable concentration
MSDS	Material safety data sheet
N/A	Not applicable
NAICS	North American Industry Classification System
ND	None detected
ng/cm²	Nanograms per square centimeter
ng/m³	Nanograms per cubic meter
NIOSH	National Institute for Occupational Safety and Health
OEL	Occupational exposure limit
OSHA	Occupational Safety and Health Administration
PBZ	Personal breathing zone
PEL	Permissible exposure limit
PPE	Personal protective equipment
PTFE	Polytetrafluoroethylene
REL	Recommended exposure limit
RH	Relative humidity
SOP	Standard operating procedure
STEL	Short-term exposure limit
THC	Tetrahydrocannabinol
TLV®	Threshold limit value
TWA	Time-weighted average
VAV	Variable air volume
VOC	Volatile organic compound
WEEL™	Workplace environmental exposure level

The National Institute for Occupational Safety and Health (NIOSH) received an employer request for a health hazard evaluation at a police department in Kentucky. The employer submitted the request because employees working in a vault used to store drug evidence were experiencing health symptoms.

What NIOSH Did

- We evaluated the drug vault in December 2009 and again in July 2010.
- We held confidential medical interviews with employees.
- We sampled the air for inorganic acids that could come from the drugs stored in the vault.
- We sampled the air for volatile organic compounds (VOCs) that could be a source of the odors in the drug vault.
- We took samples from the air and work surfaces to look for residual drug particles. Specifically we were looking for cocaine, methamphetamine, oxycodone, and tetrahydrocannabinol.
- We evaluated the ventilation in the drug vault and adjacent office area.
- We measured the temperature and relative humidity (RH) in the drug vault and adjacent office area.
- We discussed the department's medical surveillance program with the employer.
- We talked to drug vault employees about operating procedures and health and safety training.

What NIOSH Found

- Drug particles found in air and on surfaces present a potential health risk to employees.
- Levels of inorganic acids in air were well below applicable occupational exposure limits.
- The VOCs that we measured in air were components of marijuana. The low levels we measured are unlikely to cause health effects.
- Visible mold contamination was found on cardboard boxes that held plant-based drugs.
- Many employees reported a variety of health symptoms. Workplace exposures (odors, mold, and drugs) and factors unrelated to work could have contributed to these symptoms.
- The exhaust air flow rate in the drug vault was adequate. However, supply air diffusers were located near the ceiling exhaust air grills, leading to reduced ventilation effectiveness.
- The drug vault was under negative pressure relative to the adjacent rooms. The office was under negative pressure relative to the adjacent hallway. Air is drawn into rooms

under negative pressure, which helps to prevent odors and contaminants from going to other areas of the building.

- Most of the temperatures and RH levels were acceptable for thermal comfort. However, the RH levels in the drug vault during the July visit were greater than 50%, which can promote mold growth.

What Managers Can Do

- Thoroughly clean contaminated surfaces with environmentally friendly cleaners. Improve housekeeping practices to prevent future contamination of surfaces.

- Improve the organization of evidence inside the drug vault.

- Dispose of drugs more frequently to reduce the amount of material that could expose employees.

- Develop written policies and standard operating procedures (SOPs) describing work practices for handling evidence inside the drug vault. Once developed, train employees on these policies and SOPs and document the training.

- Stop using respirators in the drug vault. Respirators are not necessary if policies and procedures are in place to prevent the release of drug particles into the environment.

- Use the drying chamber to remove moisture from plant-based drugs, store these drugs in sealed plastic bags, and maintain RH levels below 50%.

- Modify the existing supply and exhaust ventilation to more efficiently remove and dilute odor-causing compounds.

- Make sure employees receive all elements of the medical surveillance program.

- Start a health and safety committee. This committee should have management and employee representatives who meet regularly to address health and safety concerns.

What Employees Can Do

- Attend training on policies and SOPs when offered.

- Wear nitrile gloves when handling evidence. Avoid skin contact with marijuana plants and other drugs to reduce the potential for allergic reactions.

- Report symptoms related to work and safety concerns to a supervisor.

- Participate in the health and safety committee.

Summary

NIOSH evaluated health symptoms and potential chemical exposures among police officers who worked inside a vault used to store drug evidence. Drug particles, such as cocaine, methamphetamine, and oxycodone, were found in the air and on work surfaces. Several recommendations are provided to improve working conditions and minimize drug exposures.

In November 2009, NIOSH received an HHE request from a police department in Kentucky. The request concerned possible health effects from working inside a vault used to store drug evidence, including marijuana, cocaine, methamphetamine, and oxycodone. We conducted evaluations in December 2009 and July 2010.

We held confidential interviews with 14 employees to learn about their health and workplace concerns. We observed work processes, practices and workplace conditions. We took area and PBZ air samples for inorganic acids, VOCs, and drug particles, and work surface samples for drug particle contamination. We also evaluated the supply and exhaust ventilation systems inside the drug vault and adjacent office area and measured the temperature and RH levels in these areas.

The air concentrations of inorganic acids inside the drug vault were well below applicable OELs. The primary VOCs we identified in the drug vault were terpenes. Terpenes are chemicals produced by plants, including marijuana, that contribute to their taste and smell. The low levels we measured are unlikely to cause health effects. However, some individuals are particularly sensitive to strong odors. Only methamphetamine particles were detected in the area air samples, while all the drugs (cocaine, methamphetamine, oxycodone, and THC) were measured in some of the PBZ and surface samples. Of the compounds we measured, drug particles probably present the greatest potential health risk because of their physiological and neurological effects.

Employees reported a variety of nonspecific health symptoms, with upper respiratory symptoms, headache, eye irritation, and skin rash most commonly reported. Limited evidence exists linking low levels of indirect drug exposures to acute or chronic health effects. Nevertheless, it is possible that the drug exposures we measured could have contributed to some of the reported symptoms. These symptoms can also be caused by a variety of other occupational (e.g., odors, mold, poor indoor environmental quality, and stress) and nonoccupational factors.

The general exhaust ventilation in the drug vault was adequate for gases and vapors based on the recommended minimum exhaust rate for chemical storage rooms. However, the ceiling-mounted exhaust air grills were near the supply air diffusers, leading to short-circuiting (a situation where supply air is immediately exhausted) and reduced ventilation effectiveness. Although temperature and

Health Hazard Evaluation Report 2010-0017-3133

SUMMARY
(CONTINUED)

RH levels inside the drug vault and office were acceptable for thermal comfort of employees, RH levels above 50% measured during our July visit could promote mold growth. We found visible mold contamination on cardboard boxes used for storing plant-based drugs.

We recommend that the employer develop written policies and SOPs to ensure health and safety for employees working inside the drug vault. Employees should be trained on these policies and SOPs, and all training should be documented. All drug vault employees should participate in the medical surveillance program and wear recommended personal protective equipment. If the recommendations provided in this report are implemented, the use of respirators is not necessary inside the drug vault. A drying chamber should be used to remove moisture from plant-based drugs; these drugs should be sealed in plastic bags to prevent off-gassing. Simple modification of the existing supply and exhaust ventilation systems will improve the mixing of air and removal and dilution of the odor-causing compounds. Reducing odors may help reduce the incidence of reported symptoms. In addition, surfaces that are contaminated with drug particles should be thoroughly cleaned. Once cleaned, the recommendations we provide should help control further contamination.

Keywords: NAICS 922120 (Police Protection), drugs, drug vault, drug storage, evidence, police, narcotics, cocaine, marijuana, methamphetamine, oxycodone, surface contamination

INTRODUCTION

In November 2009, NIOSH received an HHE request from management at a police department in Kentucky. The request concerned workplace exposures and health effects among police officers who worked inside the vault used to store drug evidence. We conducted evaluations on December 16, 2009, and July 12–14, 2010.

Various drugs were stored inside the drug vault, including the cannabis marijuana, the stimulants cocaine and methamphetamine, and the narcotics heroin and oxycodone. Potential exposures included drug particles, mold from marijuana plants, chemicals used in the manufacture of drugs, and chemicals used to mask the odor of drugs. At the time of the request, two drug vault employees were experiencing health problems they believed were related to working inside the drug vault. The problems listed on the request included nosebleeds, respiratory issues, skin rashes, "memory fog," fatigue, anxiety, vision problems, burning eyes, and facial twitching. These employees were assigned to another department before our evaluation.

Prior to our evaluation, employees at the police department filed a complaint with the Kentucky Labor Cabinet, Occupational Safety and Health Program. An industrial hygienist from the Kentucky Labor Cabinet conducted indoor and outdoor area air sampling for mold and PBZ air sampling for chlorine, ethyl ether, VM&P naphtha, benzene, xylene, and toluene. The area air sampling results revealed the presence of a specific type of mold (Chaetomium) only on the indoor sample. Chaetomium is commonly found in soil and decaying plant matter. The boxed marijuana plants were likely the source of this type of mold. The PBZ air sampling results were all below the detection limits and hence, well below the applicable OELs. On the basis of these findings, the Kentucky Labor Cabinet, Occupational Safety and Health Program recommended a "drying room" to dehydrate incoming plants before packaging.

At the time of our July 2010 evaluation three employees worked inside the drug vault. The drug vault employees had a variety of duties including receipt, storage, and retrieval of drug evidence; transport of drug evidence; maintenance of inventory; and retrieving evidence for disposal. They could spend several hours per day inside the drug vault storing or retrieving evidence. The marijuana plants were typically stored in ventilated cardboard boxes. Dried marijuana leaves and other drugs were typically sealed in plastic bags, which were placed in evidence envelopes or cardboard boxes. The boxes containing drugs were stacked to the ceiling during our evaluation (Figure 1). Procedures for handling and storing drugs may have changed over time. This is meaningful because drugs are often held as evidence for a decade or longer.

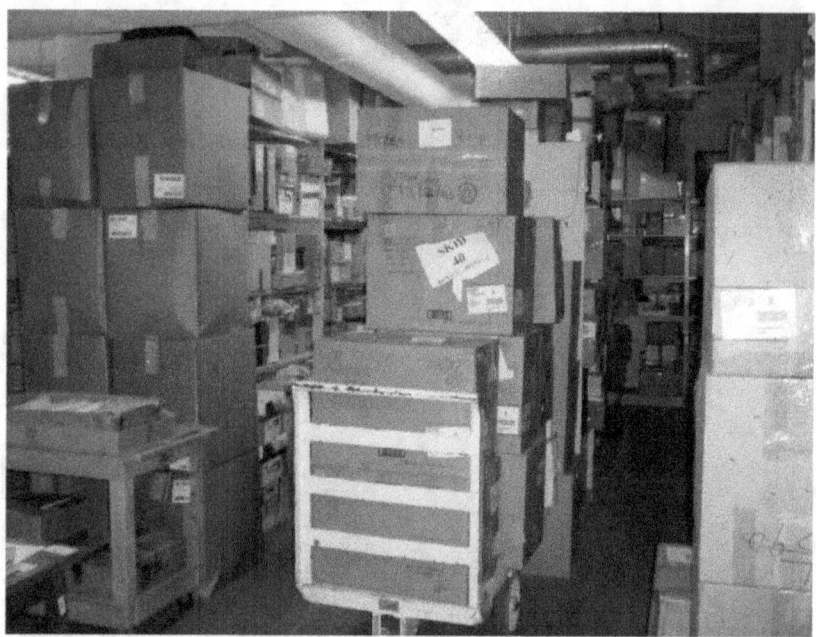

Figure 1. Interior of the drug vault showing boxes stacked to the ceiling.

The drug vault employees were required to wear NIOSH-approved Moldex (Culver City, California) elastomeric half-mask air purifying respirators (8000 series) with organic vapor cartridges (8100 series) when working in the drug vault. Although no formal written respiratory protection program had been developed, the drug vault employees were fit tested for wearing these respirators, trained on the maintenance and storage of these respirators, and were included in the medical surveillance program. Prior to our evaluation, the inventory of evidence took place inside the drug vault. At the time of the evaluation, employees used carts to bring drug evidence into the office area for inventory thereby limiting the time spent in the drug vault. Vans or trucks with lockable beds were used to transport drug evidence.

The drug vault was a 1725 ft^2-concrete block room with a 12.5-foot ceiling inside a warehouse. It could be accessed through locked doors from either the storage room or office. The office was a 200 ft^2-room with a 12.5-foot ceiling. The drug vault employees had workstations in the office area. Figure 2 shows the HVAC mechanical plan of the drug vault and adjacent areas. VAV boxes controlled the flow of conditioned air to the drug vault and office. By design, the drug vault was to receive 1445 cfm of conditioned air (no minimum), and the office was to receive 145 cfm of conditioned air (with a minimum set point of 75 cfm). The designed ratio of outdoor air to recirculated air supplied to the VAV boxes in the drug vault and office was 40%. The exhaust system was designed to remove 2800 cfm of air from the drug vault and 150 cfm of air from the office. The exhausted airflow from both areas was nearly doubled between our first and second evaluations by adding a more powerful motor for the fan. In addition, two vents were added to exhaust more air from the middle of the drug vault, and an opening was installed on the northwest wall separating the drug vault from the hallway to provide make-up air to the drug vault.

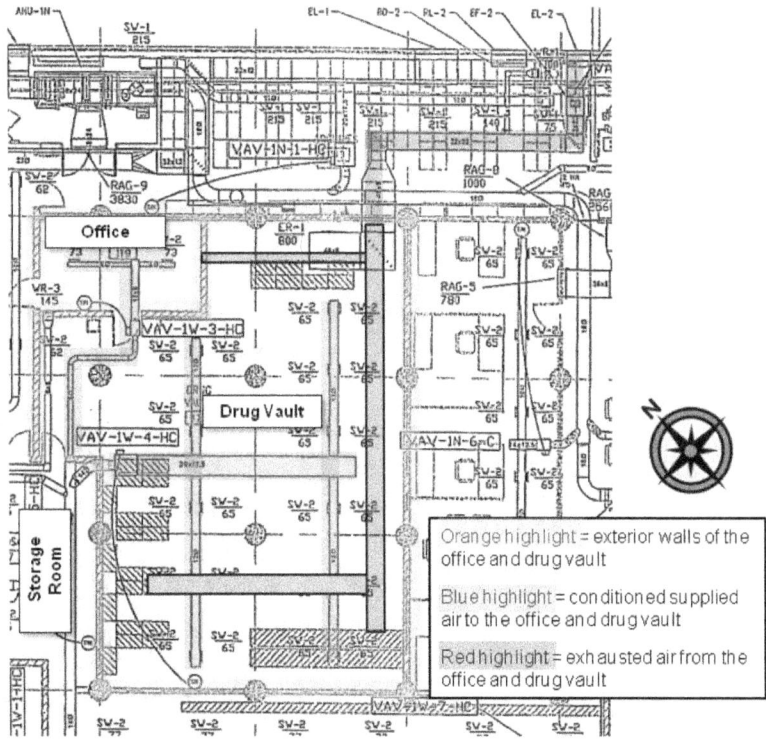

Figure 2. Floor plan showing the drug vault and adjacent areas as well as the HVAC supply ducts and exhaust ventilation ducts.

Assessment

We interviewed employees, conducted air sampling, and evaluated the ventilation system in the drug vault and office (the areas where the drug vault employees spent most of their workday). We invited all employees working in the drug vault and in the adjacent storage room to participate in confidential employee interviews. We asked about current job tasks, procedures for handling drug evidence, acute and chronic health symptoms potentially associated with exposure to drugs, PPE use, and workplace health and safety training. We reviewed the OSHA Form 300 Log of Work-Related Injuries and Illnesses for 2009.

During the December 2009 visit, we conducted PBZ and area air sampling for VOCs and inorganic acids during a single workday. Area air samples were collected inside the drug vault, inside the office, and near the HVAC outdoor air intake. PBZ air samples were collected on a drug vault employee. VOCs were sampled because a strong odor existed in the drug vault. We used a qualitative VOC analysis to identify vapors and gases. We also sampled the air for inorganic acids (hydrochloric, hydrobromic, hydrofluoric, nitric, sulfuric, and phosphoric acids) because investigators in a previous HHE at another facility had found low levels of hydrofluoric, hydrochloric, and sulfuric acid inside an evidence room containing drugs [NIOSH 1999].

During the July 2010 visit, we collected seven PBZ and six area air samples for specific drugs (methamphetamine, cocaine, oxycodone, and THC) during 3 consecutive workdays. PBZ samples were collected from three drug vault employees, and area air samples were collected inside the drug vault and office. We collected samples from various surfaces such as door handles, carts, computer mice, and shelving using swabs prewetted with sampling buffer; these samples were also analyzed for the aforementioned drugs. The air and surface sampling methods we used are intended to quantify drug particles, not gases or vapors.

We evaluated the ventilation in the drug vault and office by measuring the airflow rates in the HVAC supply ducts and exhaust ventilation ducts with a pitot tube. In addition, we used ventilation smoke tubes to assess the capture efficiency of the exhaust system and determine pressure differentials between the drug vault and adjacent areas. We measured temperature and RH inside the drug vault and office during both visits. More detailed information on the sampling methods and ventilation assessment is provided in Appendix A. Information on OELs and potential health effects for the chemicals we monitored are provided in Appendix B.

Although drug vault employees expressed concern about mold exposure, we did not sample for mold for three reasons: (1) mold is ubiquitous in the indoor and outdoor environments; thus, the presence of mold in air is not unusual and does not necessarily represent a hazardous condition, (2) mold was clearly visible on boxes and other packages containing marijuana plants; hence, air sampling would only confirm what we already know from observation, and (3) the Kentucky Labor Cabinet had previously sampled for and documented mold in the indoor air.

RESULTS

Employee Interviews

We conducted confidential health interviews with 14 employees, 11 during the December 2009 site visit and three during the July 2010 site visit. Of the 11 employees interviewed in December 2009, nine had current or prior drug vault work experience, while two worked in the storage room. All three employees working in the drug vault during our July 2010 evaluation were interviewed. The average age of employees interviewed was 40 years, and most (10 of 14) were male. Average length of employment with the department was 13 years; average length of employment for current drug vault employees was 2 years. Of the 12 employees with current or prior drug vault experience, most typically worked 40 hours a week with occasional overtime (approximately 1 day per month) if they had to prepare evidence for a court case.

The most common symptoms reported by the employees working in the drug vault and storage room were upper respiratory ailments such as sinus congestion, cough, and runny nose (reported by nine employees) and headache (reported by seven employees). All of the employees interviewed reported a strong odor that they described as the odor of "marijuana, vitamins, and other chemicals" in the drug vault; five employees attributed recurring headaches to these odors. Four employees reported olfactory fatigue, the temporary inability to distinguish a particular odor after prolonged exposure. Employees interviewed in July 2010 were new to the drug vault and were not interviewed during the December 2009 site visit.

Employees interviewed during the December 2009 site visit reported a wider variety of symptoms than those during the July 2010 site visit. One or more of the three employees interviewed during the July site visit reported eye irritation, headache, and upper respiratory symptoms. Of the nine employees interviewed in December 2009 with past experience in the drug vault, eight reported upper respiratory symptoms; seven reported headaches; five reported eye irritation; three reported skin rashes; three reported fatigue; three reported neurologic symptoms such as dizziness, tremors, visual disturbances, and short term memory loss; and one reported intermittent nosebleeds that they attributed to work in the drug vault.

Two of the employees with past work experience in the drug vault who reported skin rash described it as "breaking out in hives" that resolved after taking oral Benadryl®. Concerns about health effects from dermal exposure to drugs while packaging drug evidence in the storage room and when handling broken packaging in the drug vault were reported. Concerns about long-term chronic health effects such as cancer and other unknown health effects were expressed.

Along with health symptoms, other work-related issues were raised during the interviews, including lack of safety and health communication by the employer, insufficient training on PPE use, and need for improved housekeeping to minimize slips and trips while retrieving evidence. The OSHA Log of Illness and Injury from 2009 contained two entries for the storage room: one for sprains/strains and one for pneumonia.

Air Sampling for Inorganic Acids, VOCs, and Drugs

The MDCs and MQCs for the compounds we sampled were calculated by dividing the analytical method limit of detection and limit of quantitation for each compound by the average volume of air sampled. The MDCs and MQCs represent the smallest air concentrations that could have been detected or quantified, respectively, on the basis of volume of air sampled. MDCs and MQCs were calculated separately for PBZ and area air samples.

During the December 2009 visit, the PBZ concentrations of hydrochloric, nitric, sulfuric, hydrobromic, hydrofluoric, and phosphoric acids were ND (below their respective MDCs of 0.02, 0.02, 0.04, 0.02, 0.01, and 0.04 mg/m^3). Consequently, inhalation exposures to inorganic acids did not exceed the applicable OELs.

Hydrochloric, nitric, and sulfuric acids were measured at concentrations above their MDCs in the area air samples. These area

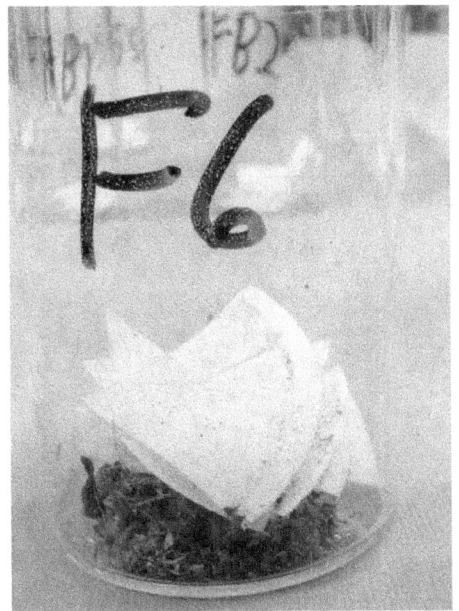

Figure 3. Particles > 1 mm in diameter that were collected on a PBZ filter sample.

air concentrations are presented in Table 1, along with the MDCs, MQCs, and applicable OELs. All the inorganic acid concentrations were well below the applicable OELs. Concentrations between the MDC and MQC are listed in Table 1 and subsequent tables in parentheses to indicate that there is more uncertainty associated with these values than with concentrations above the MQC.

Compared to the VOCs detected outdoors (near the HVAC outdoor air intake), we found relatively higher levels of various terpenes (alpha-pinene, beta-pinene, myrcene, limonene, and beta-caryophyllene) in the drug vault, office, and PBZ of a drug vault employee. The qualitative data also indicate that the levels of these terpenes were higher in the drug vault than in the office. Because these sampling results are qualitative, we cannot provide air concentrations for these compounds.

The PBZ air sampling results for drug particles are provided in Table 2, and area air sampling results for drug particles are provided in Table 3. Methamphetamine was found in area and PBZ air samples at concentrations above MDCs. The other drugs were not found in the area air samples, but were found at quantifiable levels in some of the PBZ samples. According to the analytical laboratory, the PBZ air samples collected from drug vault employees 2 and 3 on July 12 and 13, 2010, contained large particles (> 1 mm in diameter) of organic matter that would not normally remain airborne (Figure 3).

Table 1. Area air concentrations of inorganic acids (mg/m³) measured in December 2009

Location	Sampling time (minutes)	Hydrochloric	Nitric	Sulfuric
Drug vault (Bin 30)	401	(0.021)	(0.011)	ND
Drug vault (Bin 53)	403	(0.024)	(0.015)	ND
Drug vault (Bin 74)	404	ND	(0.015)	(0.035)
Office	400	(0.030)	(0.011)	ND
Outdoor air intake	392	(0.022)	(0.014)	ND
MDC		0.01	0.01	0.03
MQC		0.063	0.031	0.074
NIOSH REL [NIOSH 2005]*		C 7.0	5.0 / STEL 10	1.0
OSHA PEL [NIOSH 2005]*		C 7.0	5.0	1.0
ACGIH TLV [ACGIH 2010]*		C 3.0	5.0 / C 10	0.2

*Ceiling limits are denoted with "C." Short-term exposure limits are denoted with "STEL." All other values are full work shift TWAs.

RESULTS

(CONTINUED)

Table 2. PBZ concentrations of drug particles (ng/m³) measured in July 2010

Date collected	Employee No.	Methamphetamine	Oxycodone	Cocaine	THC
7/12/2010	1	(2.2)	ND	ND	ND
	2*	11	ND	12000	> 38
	3*	ND	0.97	(47)	> 52
7/13/2010	1	5.0	ND	200	5.0
	2*	16	ND	930	> 51
	3*	28	(0.64)	3000	> 54
7/14/2010	1	(6.2)	ND	ND	ND
MDC		3	0.4	30	2
MQC		4.5	0.67	52	4.6

* These samples collected particles that are larger than those that are typically collected with our air sampling procedure. Thus, these samples may not accurately estimate the PBZ concentrations of the drugs.

Table 3. Area air concentrations of drug particles (ng/m³) measured in July 2010

Date collected	Location	Methamphetamine	Oxycodone	Cocaine	THC
7/12/2010	Office	(2.2)	ND	ND	ND
	Drug vault	3.1	ND	ND	ND
7/13/2010	Office	(1.2)	ND	ND	ND
	Drug vault	2.8	ND	ND	ND
7/14/2010	Office	(2.4)	ND	ND	ND
	Drug vault	5.2	ND	ND	ND
MDC		2	0.3	20	1.5
MQC		3.1	0.46	36	3.1

RESULTS
(CONTINUED)

Table 4. Masses of drugs on surfaces (ng/100 cm^2) in the drug vault, office, and storage room

Area	Location	Surface description	Meth*	Oxycodone	Cocaine	THC
Office	Desk of employee 1	Laminate	ND	ND	ND	ND
	Desk of employee 2	Laminate	ND	(2.1)	(330)	ND
	Top of cart used to transport evidence	Plastic	(8.2)	ND	4600	ND
	Handle of cart used to transport evidence†	Plastic	ND	3.6	1900	ND
	Computer mouse at the desk of employee 2†	Plastic	ND	ND	ND	ND
	Handle of refrigerator†	Plastic	ND	ND	(310)	ND
	Box used to hold envelopes containing evidence	Cardboard	18	ND	(370)	ND
	Handle of door between office and drug vault†	Stainless steel	ND	(2.1)	800	ND
Drug vault	3rd movable shelf from south side of the room	Steel	ND	ND	7300	ND
	Shelf 53 at the south side of the room	Steel	24	ND	920	(26)
	Storage box containing marijuana plants	Cardboard	ND	ND	ND	ND
	Large table in the center of the room	Laminate	ND	(1.9)	4800	41
	Control panel for movable shelving	Plastic	79	ND	2300	ND
	Cart for transporting evidence	Plastic	59	3.6	4300	ND
	Handle of door between drug vault and storage room†	Stainless steel	ND	3.30	(400)	ND
Storage room	Evidence shoot	Steel	49	(2.49)	980	ND
Limit of detection			6	2	300	20
Limit of quantitation			12	2.9	420	40

* Meth = methamphetamine

† The entire surface was sampled. The surface area was not determined, and hence, may not be 100 square centimeters.

Currently, no OELs exist for the drugs we sampled, most likely because airborne exposures to drugs are unusual in most occupations. The one exception is oxycodone, a commonly prescribed narcotic that could become aerosolized in the pharmaceutical and healthcare industries. According to the MSDS published by Purdue Pharma L.P. (Cranbury, New Jersey) for OxyContin® tablets, workplace exposures to oxycodone (free base) dusts should be kept below the manufacturer's OEL of 40,000 ng/m^3 [Purdue Pharma 2010]. The area and PBZ concentrations of oxycodone we measured were well below these manufacturer's guidelines.

Surface Sampling for Drugs

The surface sampling results for each drug sampled are presented in Table 4. Quantifiable levels of methamphetamine, cocaine, oxycodone, and THC were found at various locations in the drug vault and office. Cocaine was found in the highest quantities (ranging up to 7300 ng/100 cm^2) on surfaces that were sampled. No federal standards exist for drug surface contamination. However, several states have established feasibility-based surface contamination limits when remediating clandestine laboratories for methamphetamine ranging from 100 ng/100 cm^2 to 500 ng/100 cm^2 [NAMSDL 2008]. The range of methamphetamine contamination that we measured (ND to 79 ng/100 cm^2) was below these limits.

Assessment of Ventilation, Temperature, and Humidity

Figure 4 shows the locations where pitot tube traverses were performed to measure airflow in the supply and exhaust ducts. The supply and exhaust airflow rates are presented in Table 5. Certification measurements of the exhaust system recorded on June 23, 2010, are provided for comparison against our measurements recorded on July 13, 2010. The measurements we recorded were similar to the certification measurements.

Under its current design and operation, the exhaust system in the drug vault removed 1.6 cfm/ft^2, resulting in approximately 7.6 air changes per hour. Because more air was exhausted from the drug vault (2,720 cfm) than that which the HVAC system supplied to the vault (1,713 cfm), the drug vault was under negative pressure relative to its adjacent space (i.e., storage room, office, and hallway). This means that air from adjacent areas flowed into the drug vault. Approximately 850 cfm of make-up air came through the ventilation hole in the northwest wall of the drug vault. The rest of the make-up air most likely came through leaks around the doors or any cracks in the drug vault walls.

To further assess pressure differentials, we used ventilation smoke tubes to generate smoke along the perimeter of the door connecting the drug vault and office. We observed smoke being drawn from the office into the drug vault, demonstrating that the vault was under negative pressure. Using the same method, we found that the office was under negative pressure relative to the hallway. It is ideal for the drug vault and office to be under negative pressure relative to adjacent areas. Also using smoke tubes, we identified four locations (Figure 4) where an HVAC supply diffuser was so close to an exhaust grill that supply air was immediately exhausted from the room. This phenomenon, called short-circuiting, reduces the effectiveness of the ventilation.

The temperature and RH measurements made in the drug vault and office during our evaluation are summarized in Table 6. As expected, RH levels were higher in July than in December. The temperature and RH were slightly more variable in the office than in the drug vault. The thermostats in both locations could only be increased or decreased by 2°F from a set point specified by facilities management.

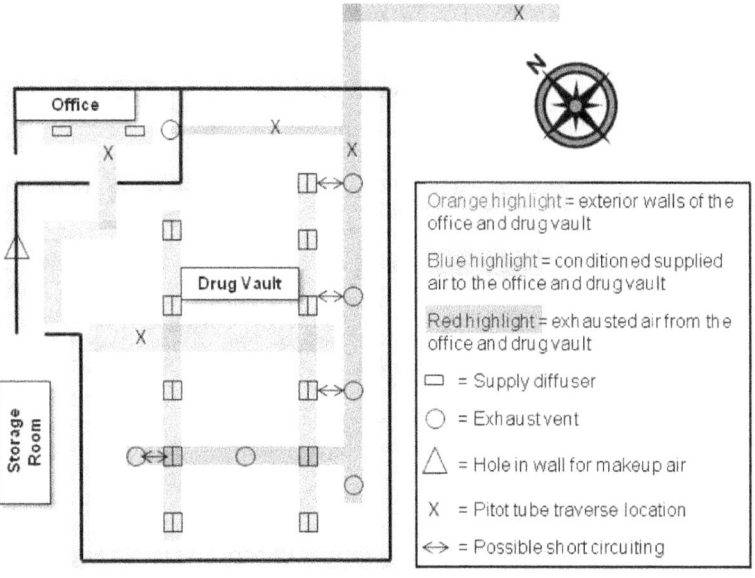

Figure 4. Supply and exhaust ventilation in the drug vault and office.

Table 5. Supply and exhaust airflow rates in the drug vault and office

HVAC component	Airflow rate (cfm)		
	Design	Certification measurement on 6/23/10	NIOSH measurement on 7/13/10
Drug vault supply	1,445	N/A	1,713
Drug vault make-up air (through 1.7 ft² vent to adjacent hallway)*	N/A	N/A	850
Office supply	145 / 75 minimum	N/A	122
Total exhaust (negative pressure side of exhaust fan)	2,972	2,926	2,944
Drug vault exhaust	2,822	2,786	2,720
NE branch exhaust	2,522	2,535	N/A
NW branch exhaust	300	251	N/A
Office exhaust	150	132	103

* Recorded using a hot wire anemometer. All other airflows were determined using pitot-tubes.

Table 6. Temperature and humidity levels measured in the drug vault and office

Location	Date sampled	Sampling time (hours)	Temperature (°F)		RH (%)	
			Mean	Range	Mean	Range
Office	12/16/2009	8	74	72–75	9.2	7.2–9.8
Drug vault	12/16/2009	8	74	73–75	10.5	8.8–11
Office	7/12/2010 to 7/14/2010	52	73	72–75	53	49–58
Drug vault	7/12/2010 to 7/14/2010	52	69	68–70	64	61–66

Other Observations

During our December 2009 visit, we observed problems associated with storage procedures and housekeeping practices. We noted a bottle of codeine that was leaking onto the floor, boxes of drugs stacked to the ceiling, dust and debris on various surfaces inside the drug vault (Figure 5), and trash cans that had not been emptied for several days. By our July 2010 visit, several changes had been made to improve drug handling procedures. For example, drug evidence was sealed in plastic before packaging in an envelope, and packages leaking liquid drugs were placed into plastic bags. In addition, a vacuum containing a HEPA air filter and a chamber

(Safestore chemical storage cabinet, Air Science USA LLC, Fort Myers, Florida) for drying plants had been purchased. However, the HEPA vacuum and drying chamber had not yet been used.

We also observed problems during the July 2010 visit. Some drug vault employees wearing elastomeric half-mask respirators had facial hair that could interfere with the seal of the respirator. Thin plastic garbage bags containing prescription drugs collected from the public for proper disposal had torn. The van used to transport drug evidence to and from the police department had loose plant material (presumably from marijuana evidence that spilled on the floor of the vehicle) (Figure 6).

Shortly after our July 2010 visit, a drying chamber was installed just outside the drug vault in the storage room. The drying chamber was not ducted to the outdoors, but the exhausted air was filtered using organic vapor and particulate air filters. The drying chamber was used to dry marijuana plants. Large amounts of these plants were then stored in cardboard boxes, and small amounts were stored in paper envelopes inside the drug vault. The drug vault employees reported that use of the drying chamber has helped reduce the intensity of "marijuana" odors inside the drug vault.

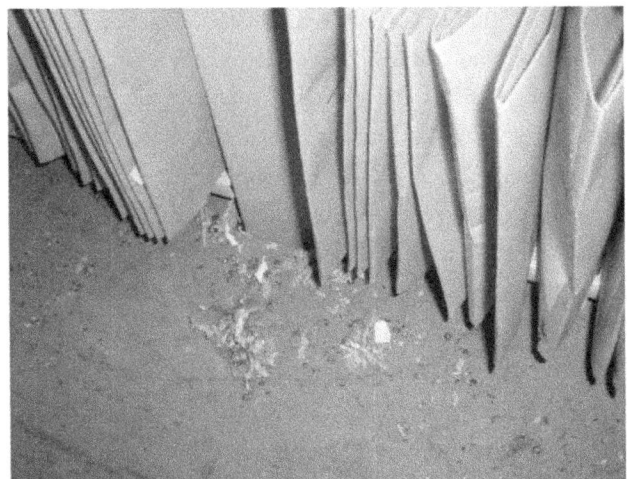

Figure 5. Debris on the surface of shelving used to store envelopes containing drug evidence.

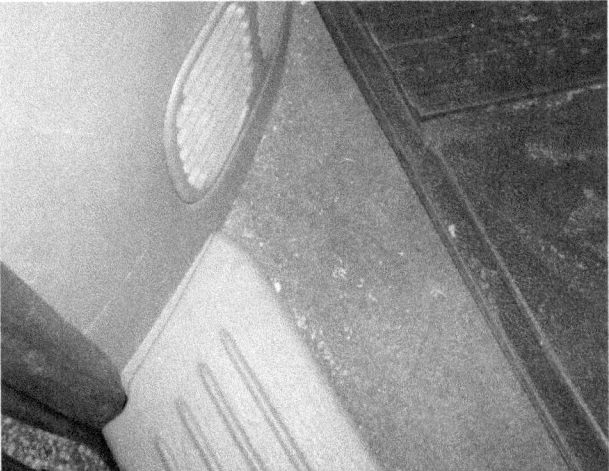

Figure 6. Debris on the floor of the van used to transport drug evidence.

DISCUSSION

Potential Exposures

A previous HHE conducted in an evidence room containing drugs found low levels of hydrofluoric, hydrochloric, and sulfuric acids [NIOSH 1999]. Sulfuric acid can be used in clandestine methamphetamine laboratories, and hydrochloric acid can be used in the production of methamphetamine, cocaine, and phencyclidine [NIOSH 1999]. These acids could therefore be present as an impurity in these drugs. However, the levels of acids we measured in the indoor air samples were well below applicable OELs. Further, the levels in the drug vault were comparable to the levels measured in the outdoor air samples, suggesting that the drug vault was not the source for the acids.

According to the qualitative VOC sample results, elevated levels of various terpenes (alpha-pinene, beta-pinene, myrcene, limonene, and beta-caryophyllene) were found in the drug vault, office, and PBZ of a drug vault employee. These compounds are common volatile constituents of marijuana [Lai et al. 2008] and likely contributed to the "marijuana" odors in the drug vault and office. Terpenes are also commonly used in cleaners. However, cleaners were probably not the source of these odors because the drug vault employees had not recently cleaned inside the drug vault. Of the terpenes we measured, only limonene has an OEL (AIHA WEEL of 170 mg/m^3 as an 8-hour TWA), which is intended to prevent adverse affects to the liver [AIHA 2010]. Because the sampling method we used was qualitative, we do not know the exact concentration of limonene in the drug vault. However, according to the analytical laboratory, nanogram levels of limonene (and other terpenes) were collected on the VOC samples. Thus, the air concentrations of limonene were probably at least three orders of magnitude lower than the AIHA WEEL. These low levels of terpenes are unlikely to cause adverse health effects.

Quantifiable levels of various drugs were measured in the PBZs of the drug vault employees. Only methamphetamine was quantified in the area air samples. Unlike the VOCs that are present as gases and vapors, the drugs we sampled exist as particles. Drug particles must be agitated and/or circulated in the air for employees to be exposed via the inhalation route. The particles on the air samples collected from drug vault employees 2 and 3 on July 12, 2010, and July 13, 2010, were much larger (>1 mm in diameter) than the size of particles that are normally collected on these air filters. Therefore, a problem with the collection of these air samples may have led to an overestimate of PBZ concentrations of the drugs.

The PBZ concentrations of methamphetamine, oxycodone, and THC ranged from ND to >54 ng/m^3, while the PBZ concentrations of cocaine ranged from ND to 12,000 ng/m^3. Even though some of the air samples may have overestimated the PBZ concentrations of the drugs, the concentrations we measured were relatively low. For perspective, most OELs for particles are expressed in mg/m^3, and drug users usually take several milligrams of a drug [Gable 2004]; a nanogram is one million times smaller than a milligram. Low exposures, however, do not necessarily equate to safe and healthy conditions because some compounds can elicit health effects at very small doses. Purdue-Pharma L.P. established an OEL for oxycodone of 40,000 ng/m^3 to prevent respiratory irritation or allergies [Purdue Pharma 2010]. The oxycodone levels we measured in air were well below this OEL. We could not find a published OEL for cocaine; however, the airborne levels of cocaine were considerably higher than any other drug we measured.

The surface sampling we conducted confirmed the presence of drug particles on surfaces in the drug vault and office where hand contact is likely (e.g., handle of cart, handle of refrigerator, surface of desk, evidence shoot, etc.). Particles can be transferred from surfaces to hands, and in the absence of adequate hand-washing, can then be transferred from hands to the mouth when employees eat or smoke in the workplace. This represents a possible route of exposure (ingestion) to drugs. If employees were to rub their eyes, drugs could be transferred to the eyes. Airborne drug particles could also contact the eyes. In both cases, eye irritation is possible. Skin irritation could also occur from drugs contacting the skin. Bringing low levels of drug contamination home is also a possibility.

Methamphetamine levels measured on surfaces were below the lowest feasibility-based surface contamination limits (100 ng/100 cm^2). Levels of cocaine collected in 9 of 16 samples, on the other hand, exceeded the highest surface contamination limit for methamphetamine (500 ng/100 cm^2) and the largest amount of cocaine measured on a surface was 14 times this limit. Because cocaine and methamphetamine are both stimulants [DEA 2010], the levels of cocaine surface contamination we measured could present a hazard to the drug vault employees and therefore warrants remediation.

Ventilation, Temperature, and Humidity

According to ANSI/ASHRAE Standard 62.1-2010 [ASHRAE 2010a], a minimum outdoor air rate of 34 cfm should be supplied to the office (based on three person occupancy and zone air distribution effectiveness of 0.8). If the supply air contained 40% outdoor air as currently scheduled, then approximately 50 cfm of outdoor air was supplied to the office when the VAV box was at maximum flow (122 cfm, as measured) and 30 cfm of outdoor air was supplied to the office when the VAV box was at minimum flow (75 cfm, as designed).

ASHRAE does not provide specific exhaust ventilation recommendations for drug vaults or evidence rooms other than that they should be kept under negative pressure [ASHRAE 2007a]. However, in a previous HHE report, investigators recommended 6 air changes per hour for an evidence room containing drugs and other chemicals [NIOSH 1999]. This recommendation was based on the ASHRAE guidelines for chemical laboratories [ASHRAE 2007b]. According to the International Association for Identification safety guidelines [IAI 2004], areas where drugs and other chemicals are maintained should have constant exhaust ventilation resulting in a minimum of 7 air changes per hour. According to our measurements, the drug vault had about 7.6 air changes per hour (based on the exhaust rate). However, the number of air changes per hour is influenced greatly by the size of the room and does not account for contaminant generation rate or the mixing of air in the room [ASHRAE 2007c]. Uniform mixing occurs when the supply air is instantly and evenly distributed throughout a space [ACGIH 2007]. Air mixing in the drug vault was not uniform because the ceiling-mounted supply air diffusers and exhaust air grills were near each other. We identified four areas where the exhaust air grills were too close to the supply air diffusers, resulting in short-circuiting—a situation where supply air is immediately exhausted. Short-circuiting reduces the effective exhaust rate of contaminants or nuisance odors.

ASHRAE recommends minimum exhaust rates for different occupancy categories [ASHRAE 2010a]. A drug vault is not identified specifically, but is most similar to a chemical storage room because both contain potentially hazardous substances in sealed containers. The most hazardous airborne contaminants we found in the drug vault were drug particles. General exhaust ventilation is intended for gases and vapors but not for particles. The gases and vapors we measured in the drug vault were volatile constituents of marijuana. Most of these compounds are not considered hazardous. Nevertheless, the exhaust rate in the drug vault (1.6 cfm/ft²) was greater than the minimum exhaust rate for chemical storage rooms (1.5 cfm/ft²). Increasing this exhaust rate further will not necessarily reduce the "marijuana" odors because the emitted compounds have very low odor thresholds. Isolating marijuana to its own ventilated room or packaging marijuana to contain the off-gassing chemicals will do more to reduce odors than increasing the general exhaust ventilation.

As recommended by ASHRAE [ASHRAE 2007a], the drug vault was under constant negative pressure relative to the adjacent areas. Thus, if the doors remain closed nuisance odors should not readily migrate to the office where the drug vault employees spent most of their workday. In addition, the office was under negative pressure relative to the adjacent hallway, which is appropriate because packages containing drugs are handled inside the office.

ASHRAE recommends keeping evidence vaults at 72°F–74°F and 30% RH in the winter and no more than 50% RH in the summer [ASHRAE 2007a]. We measured RH levels below this range in the winter and above this range in the summer. Maintaining RH levels below 50% reduces the potential for mold growth. RH levels far below 30% may dry out skin and mucous membranes, but we typically do not advise adding moisture to indoor air (humidification). Most of the temperature and RH levels we measured were within the acceptable range of operative temperature and humidity for thermal comfort as specified in ANSI/ASHRAE Standard 55-2010 [ASHRAE 2010b]. However, the temperature and RH levels in the drug vault from July 12–14. 2010, were below the acceptable range for persons wearing clothing made of thin materials (typical of warmer months). Moreover, the employees felt that they did not have sufficient control over the climate in the office and drug vault.

Health Symptoms

Acute and chronic health effects from exposures to very low levels of the types of drugs sampled in this evaluation are not well understood. Information that is available about the mechanism of action of these drugs and their health effects at higher doses

Discussion
(continued)

is found in Appendix B. Multiple factors could contribute to the nonspecific symptoms reported by employees. These factors are difficult to sort out to assess their individual contributions to reported symptoms. The factors include mold exposure, poor indoor environmental quality, discomfort due to fluctuations in temperature and humidity, odors, and stress. Some employees may be more sensitive to these factors than others, thus are more likely to report symptoms. Although acute and chronic health effects from the very low levels of drugs found in the evaluation appear unlikely, we cannot definitively state that they did not contribute in part to reported symptoms. Additionally, drug exposures likely vary over time and may be higher during periods of increased workload and evidence processing, during drug transport and disposal operations, or when large amounts of inventory are in the drug vault.

Skin rashes were reported by three drug vault employees. Several case reports in the scientific literature report dermatitis from occupational exposure and handling of Cannabis (marijuana) plants and materials, with symptoms increasing over time with ongoing exposure [Majmudar et al. 2006; Williams et al. 2008].

Conclusions

Exposures to the drug particles found in this occupational setting probably present the greatest potential health risk given their well-known neurological and physiological effects at relatively high doses. However, the exposure levels we measured were low. Even though the reported symptoms could have been the result of various occupational and nonoccupational factors, it is wise to reduce exposures to all drug particles as much as feasible. Implementation of the recommendations below will help limit exposures to drug particles, chemical odors, and mold, and should help improve general indoor environmental quality and reported health symptoms. Some individuals may continue to report symptoms due to pre-existing medical conditions, nonoccupational exposures, and personal sensitivity; these cases should be handled on a case-by-case basis between the employee(s), management, and their healthcare provider.

On the basis of our findings, we recommend the actions listed below to create a more healthful workplace. We encourage the police department to use a labor-management health and safety committee or working group to discuss the recommendations in this report and develop an action plan. Those involved in the work can best set priorities and assess the feasibility of our recommendations for the specific situation at this drug vault. Our recommendations are based on the hierarchy of controls approach (Appendix B: Occupational Exposure Limits and Health Effects). This approach groups actions by their likely effectiveness in reducing or removing hazards. In most cases, the preferred approach is to eliminate hazardous materials or processes and install engineering controls to reduce exposure or shield employees. Until such controls are in place, or if they are not effective or feasible, administrative measures and/or personal protective equipment may be needed.

Elimination and Substitution

Elimination or substitution of a toxic/hazardous process material is a highly effective means for reducing hazards. Incorporating this strategy into the design or development phase of a project, commonly referred to as "prevention through design," is most effective because it reduces the need for additional controls in the future.

1. Dispose of drugs more frequently to reduce the amount of material in the drug vault that could off-gas and expose employees.

Engineering Controls

Engineering controls reduce exposures to employees by removing the hazard from the process or placing a barrier between the hazard and the employee. Engineering controls are very effective at protecting employees without placing primary responsibility of implementation on the employee.

1. Continue to dry marijuana and other plant-based drugs prior to storage to reduce odors and mold growth.

2. Replace the organic vapor and particulate filters in the drying chamber according to manufacturer's guidelines or

more frequently if odors are detected in the drying chamber exhaust. Failure to do so could result in the release of VOCs from the plant-based drugs into the indoor environment.

3. Move the drying chamber into the drug vault to prevent the odors and particles from entering the HVAC system. Another option would be to connect the drying chamber exhaust directly to the exhaust system for the drug vault. This may eliminate the need for organic vapor and particulate filters but would require capital costs associated with the modification.

4. Relocate either the supply air diffuser or exhaust air grill in the four locations (Figure 4) where they are too close to one another inside the drug vault. Alternatively, install a diffuser style that will direct the supply air away from the exhaust inlet. This will prevent short-circuiting and improve the performance of the ventilation system.

5. After drying plant-based drugs, store the plants in sealed plastic bags to minimize the release of VOCs into the environment. If these drugs continue to be stored in ventilated cardboard boxes, place them an enclosed area of the drug vault with exhaust ventilation. This will help contain odors to the enclosed area.

6. Continue to seal all other drugs in plastic. Seal and bubble-wrap glass containers containing drug evidence to minimize breakage. Use more durable plastic garbage bags for the collection of prescription medications. These bags will be less likely to tear, and their use will help reduce the likelihood of unintentional release of VOCs into the environment. If drug contamination is evident on existing packages, seal these packages in another plastic bag.

7. Provide conditioned air to maintain an RH at 30%–50% to the drug vault throughout the year. This will also help minimize mold growth.

8. Use a truck with a lockable bed enclosure to transport drugs to and from the police department. This will reduce employee exposures to dusts or VOCs from the drugs during transport.

Administrative Controls

Administrative controls are management-dictated work practices and policies to reduce or prevent exposures to workplace hazards. The effectiveness of administrative changes in work practices for controlling workplace hazards is dependent on management commitment and employee acceptance. Regular monitoring and reinforcement are necessary to ensure that control policies and procedures are not circumvented in the name of convenience or production.

1. Conduct a thorough cleaning of the surfaces inside the drug vault, office, and storage room where drug contamination was found (or is likely to be present). A HEPA vacuum can be used for porous surfaces and nonporous surfaces containing larger particles. Environmentally-friendly cleaners and disposable paper towels can be used for all other nonporous surfaces. Employees performing the cleaning should wear nitrile gloves or other suitable gloves as recommended by the manufacturers of the chosen cleaners.

2. Improve housekeeping practices. Empty the trash inside the drug vault daily, and vacuum the floors weekly with a HEPA vacuum. Surfaces that directly contact packages of evidence (carts, tables, etc.) should be cleaned weekly with an environmentally-friendly cleaner. Because there are no regulations regarding what can be labeled "environmentally friendly," management will need to become knowledgeable about what cleaning materials are appropriate. Useful sources of information to help select the safest products include the National Institutes of Health database at http://householdproducts.nlm.nih.gov/ and the Greenguard Environmental Institute at http://www.greenguard.org/. These housekeeping practices will help minimize the potential for exposures to drug particles and improve the air quality by reducing allergens and nuisance odors. The HEPA filter in the vacuum will need to be replaced routinely per manufacturer's specifications.

3. Improve the organization of evidence inside the drug vault. Boxes should be neatly stacked and accessible. Avoid stacking boxes to the ceiling. Use labels that have larger print and are easier to read. These procedures should ease evidence retrieval and minimize the potential for chemical exposures or injuries when trying to locate evidence.

RECOMMENDATIONS
(CONTINUED)

4. Use a cart to transport evidence packages from the drop-off bins to the drug vault. This will reduce the likelihood of dropping a package containing breakable items.

5. Wash hands thoroughly after removing gloves and before eating, drinking, or smoking to prevent potential hand to mouth transmission and ingestion of drug particles.

6. Avoid skin contact with marijuana plants and material to reduce the potential for irritation and allergic reactions.

7. Ensure that employees included in the existing medical surveillance program are receiving all elements of the program, which should include a general health questionnaire and follow up for employees who have shown health changes. If respirator use for employees continues to be required as discussed below, medical clearance specific for respirator wear is required by OSHA regulation. Spirometry (breathing test) should be conducted for employees based on a medical provider's professional opinion.

8. Continue to have employees report any adverse health symptoms to their supervisors as they occur. Employees who continue to experience symptoms should be evaluated by a healthcare provider with experience in evaluating occupational health concerns, with referral to medical specialists (i.e., dermatologist, pulmonologist) as appropriate.

9. Organize a health and safety committee consisting of management and employee representatives (including the Fraternal Order of Police) who meet regularly to address health and safety concerns.

10. Develop written policies and SOPs for the drug vault employees describing the work practices and required PPE for work involving drug evidence. Training on these policies and SOPs should be conducted and documented for drug vault employees.

Personal Protective Equipment

PPE is the least effective means for controlling employee exposures. Proper use of PPE requires a comprehensive program, and calls for a high level of employee involvement and commitment to be effective. The use of PPE requires the choice of the appropriate equipment to reduce the hazard and the development of supporting programs such as training, change-out schedules, and medical assessment if needed. PPE should not be relied upon as the sole method for limiting employee exposures. Rather, PPE should be used until engineering and administrative controls can be demonstrated to be effective in limiting exposures to acceptable levels.

1. Wear nitrile gloves when handling evidence to prevent skin exposures.

2. Stop wearing air purifying respirators when entering the drug vault. The elastomeric half-mask air purifying respirators currently provided are equipped with organic vapor cartridges that are not protective against particles; some employees had facial hair that interfered with the proper seal of these respirators. Moreover, the potential for exposure to drug particles and other contaminants will be greatly reduced by following the other recommendations provided in this report. However, if the use of respirators continues to be mandatory for work in the drug vault, then a *comprehensive* respiratory protection program should be implemented that meets the requirements of the OSHA regulations [29 CFR 1910.134]. Such a program includes training on the proper wear and maintenance of respirators, medical clearance, and respirator fit testing. If respirator use is made voluntary, then a *limited* respiratory protection program should be implemented that meets the requirements specified in paragraph (c) (2) of the OSHA regulations [29 CFR 1910.134].

REFERENCES

ACGIH [2007]. Industrial ventilation: a manual of recommended practice for design, 26th ed. Cincinnati, OH: American Conference of Governmental Industrial Hygienists (ACGIH).

ACGIH [2010]. Threshold limit values for chemical substances and physical agents and biological exposure indices. Cincinnati, OH: American Conference of Governmental Industrial Hygienists.

AIHA [2010]. Emergency Response Planning Guidelines and Worplace Environmental Exposure Levels. Fairfax, VA: American Industrial Hygiene Association (AIHA).

ASHRAE [2007a]. Justice facilities. In: 2007 ASHRAE handbook: heating, ventilating, and air-conditioning applications. Atlanta, GA: American Society of Heating, Refrigerating and Air-Conditioning Engineers, Inc.

ASHRAE [2007b]. Laboratories. In: ASHRAE handbook: heating, ventilating, and air-conditioning applications. Atlanta, GA: American Society of Heating, Refrigerating and Air-Conditioning Engineers, Inc.

ASHRAE [2007c]. Ventilation and infiltration. In: 2007 ASHRAE handbook: heating, ventilating, and air-conditioning applications. Atlanta, GA: American Society of Heating, Refrigerating and Air-Conditioning Engineers, Inc.

ASHRAE [2010a]. ANSI/ASHRAE Standard 62.1-2010: Ventilation for acceptable indoor air quality. Atlanta, GA: American Society of Heating, Refrigerating, and Air-Conditioning Engineers, Inc.

ASHRAE [2010b]. ANSI/ASHRAE Standard 55-2010: Thermal environmental conditions for human occupancy. Atlanta, GA: American Society of Heating, Refrigerating, and Air-Conditioning Engineers, Inc.

CFR. Code of Federal Regulations. Washington, DC: U.S. Government Printing Office, Office of the Federal Register.

DEA [2010]. Drug Enforcement Agency (DEA) drug information. [http://www.justice.gov/dea/pubs/abuse/index.htm]. Date accessed: May 2011.

Gable RS [2004]. Comparison of acute lethal toxicity of commonly abused psychoactive substances. Addiction 99(6):686–696.

IAI [2004]. Safety Guidelines: 2nd ed. Hollywood, FL: International Association for Identification (IAI).

Lai H, Corbin I, Almirall JR [2008]. Headspace sampling and detection of cocaine, MDMA, and marijuana via volatile markers in the presence of potential interferences by solid phase microextraction-ion mobility spectrometry (SPME-IMS). Anal Bioanal Chem 392(1-2):105–113.

Majmudar V, Azam N, Finch T [2006]. Contact urticaria to Cannabis sativa. Contact Dermatitis 54:127.

NAMSDL [2008]. State feasibility-based standards. Alexandria, VA: National Alliance for Model State Drug Laws (NAMSDL) [http://www.namsdl.org/documents/RemediationStandardChartFinal.pdf]. Date accessed: May 2011.

NIOSH [1999]. Hazard evaluation and technical assistance report: State of Iowa Division of Narcotics Enforcement, Des Moines, Iowa. By Burton NC. Cincinnati, OH: U.S. Department of Health and Human Services, Centers for Disease Control, National Institute for Occupational Safety and Health, NIOSH HETA Report No. 99-0252-2831.

NIOSH [2005]. NIOSH pocket guide to chemical hazards. Barsen ME, ed. Cincinnati, OH: U.S. Department of Health and Human Services, Centers for Disease Control and Prevention, National Institute for Occupational Safety and Health (NIOSH) Publication No. 2005-149.

Purdue Pharma [2010]. Material safety data sheet for OxyContin tablets. [http://www.purduepharma.com/MSDSs/OxyContin_binder.pdf]. Date accessed: May 2011.

Williams C, Thompstone J, Wilkinson M [2008]. Work-related contact urticaria to Cannibis sativa. Contact Dermatitis 58(1):62–63.

Air Sampling for VOCs

Area and PBZ air sampling for VOCs was conducted using thermal desorption tubes attached to SKC pocket pumps calibrated at 200 cubic centimeters per minute (SKC Inc., Eighty Four, Pennsylvania). The thermal desorption tubes contained three beds of sorbent material: (1) 90 milligrams of Carbopack™ Y, (2) 115 milligrams of Carbopack B, and (3) 150 milligrams Carboxen™. After sampling, the thermal desorption tubes were stored in a cooler and then qualitatively analyzed for various VOCs according to NIOSH Method 2549 [NIOSH 2010].

Air Sampling for Inorganic Acids

Area and PBZ air sampling for inorganic acids was conducted using SKC silica gel sorbent tubes (200 milligrams/400 milligrams with glass fiber filter plug) attached to SKC pocket pumps calibrated at 50 cubic centimeters per minute. After sampling, the silica gel tubes were stored in a cooler and then analyzed for hydrochloric, hydrobromic, hydrofluoric, nitric, sulfuric, and phosphoric acids according to NIOSH Method 7903 [NIOSH 2010].

Air and Surface Sampling for Drugs

Area and PBZ air sampling for particle phase drugs was conducted using SKC 37-mm diameter, 2-micrometer pore size PTFE filters attached to SKC Aircheck 2000 pumps calibrated at 4 liters per minute. Surface sampling for dusts containing drugs was conducted using cotton swabs prewetted with surface sampling buffer. For most sampling locations, a 10 × 10 centimeter template was placed over the surface and then the prewetted cotton swab was rubbed across the surface in one direction and again in the opposite direction (a crisscross pattern). After swabbing the surface, we broke the handle of the swab and placed the head of the swab in a vial containing 1 milliliter of buffer solution. For irregularly shaped objects (e.g., door handles, computer mice, and cart handles), we sampled the entire surface.

After sampling, the PTFE filters and swabs were stored in a cooler and then analyzed for methamphetamine, oxycodone, and THC with a fluorescence covalent microbead immunosorbent assay as described by Smith et al. in 2010 [Smith et al. 2010]. This assay was also used to analyze the samples for cocaine. A standard curve for cocaine was generated to calculate cocaine equivalent values. The values of the drugs collected from the surfaces were corrected using the surface recovery values determined previously [Smith et al. 2010]. For the air samples, extraction was done in methanol, the extraction solutions were then dried, and the residue was re-extracted with the surface sampling buffer. The detection and quantitation limits were provided for each analyte. However, because trace drugs (or interfering compounds) were identified on the field and laboratory blanks, the detection and quantitation limits were adjusted. Adjustments were made by adding the average analyte concentration measured on the field or laboratory blank (whichever was higher) to the respective detection and quantitation limits. These adjusted detection and quantitation limits were used in calculating the MDCs and MQCs.

Ventilation Assessment

A VelociCalc Plus (TSI Inc., Shoreview, Minnesota) with pitot tube attachment was used to perform pitot tube traverses in the HVAC supply ducts and exhaust ventilation ducts. Figure 4 (on page 11) shows the approximate locations where the pitot tube traverses were performed. Existing holes were used to insert the pitot tube into the ducts. The round drug vault exhaust duct (20-inch diameter) and round office exhaust duct (6-inch diameter) had two insertion points: one along the y-axis and one along the x-axis. The rectangular drug vault supply duct (17.5 × 20 inches) had five insertion points, the rectangular office supply duct (8 × 12 inches) had three insertion points, and the square exhaust duct on the negative pressure side of the fan (22 × 22 inches) had four insertion points. Measurement locations in the duct were determined using the log-linear method for round ducts and the log Chebyshev method for rectangular ducts [Burgess et al. 2004].

The velocity pressure was recorded at each measurement location. The average velocity pressure was calculated for each cross section of the duct. The velocity (feet per minute) was calculated using the following formula:

$$\text{Velocity} = 4004.4\sqrt{\text{velocity pressure}}$$

Airflow (cfm) was then calculated by multiplying the velocity (feet per minute) by the cross sectional area (ft²) of the duct.

The articulating hot-wire anemometer on the VelociCalc Plus was used to measure the airflow through the ventilation hole providing make-up air to the drug vault. Irritant smoke tubes (Gastec Corporation, Kanagawa, Japan) were used to determine pressure differentials between the drug vault and adjacent rooms. The smoke tubes were also used to identify areas where supply air diffusers and exhaust air vents were too close to each other, creating a potential for short-circuiting—a situation where supplied conditioned air is immediately exhausted from the room.

In addition, temperature and RH inside the office and drug vault were measured during both visits using a HOBO humidity and temperature data logger (Onset Computer Corporation, Pocasset, Massachusetts).

References

Burgess WA, Ellenbecker MJ, Treitman RD [2004]. Airflow measurement techniques. In: Ventilation for control of the work environment, 2nd ed. Hoboken, NJ: John Wiley & Sons.

NIOSH [2010]. NIOSH manual of analytical methods. 4th ed. Schlecht PC, O'Connor PF, eds. Cincinnati, OH: U.S. Department of Health and Human Services, Centers for Disease Control and Prevention, National Institute for Occupational Safety and Health, DHHS (NIOSH) Publication No. 94-113 (August 1994); 1st Supplement Publication 96-135, 2nd Supplement Publication 98-119, 3rd Supplement Publication 2003-154. [http://www.cdc.gov/niosh/docs/2003-154/].

Smith J, Sammons D, Robertson S, Biagini R, Snawder J [2010]. Measurement of multiple drugs in urine, water, and on surfaces using fluorescence covalent microbead immunosorbent assay. Toxicol Mech Methods 20(9):587–593.

APPENDIX B: OCCUPATIONAL EXPOSURE LIMITS AND HEALTH EFFECTS

In evaluating the hazards posed by workplace exposures, NIOSH investigators use both mandatory (legally enforceable) and recommended OELs for chemical, physical, and biological agents as a guide for making recommendations. OELs have been developed by federal agencies and safety and health organizations to prevent the occurrence of adverse health effects from workplace exposures. Generally, OELs suggest levels of exposure that most employees may be exposed to for up to 10 hours per day, 40 hours per week, for a working lifetime, without experiencing adverse health effects. However, not all employees will be protected from adverse health effects even if their exposures are maintained below these levels. A small percentage may experience adverse health effects because of individual susceptibility, a preexisting medical condition, and/or a hypersensitivity (allergy). In addition, some hazardous substances may act in combination with other workplace exposures, the general environment, or with medications or personal habits of the employee to produce adverse health effects even if the occupational exposures are controlled at the level set by the exposure limit. Also, some substances can be absorbed by direct contact with the skin and mucous membranes in addition to being inhaled, which contributes to the individual's overall exposure.

Most OELs are expressed as a TWA exposure. A TWA refers to the average exposure during a normal 8- to 10-hour workday. Some chemical substances and physical agents have recommended STEL or ceiling values where adverse health effects are caused by exposures over a short period. Unless otherwise noted, the STEL is a 15-minute TWA exposure that should not be exceeded at any time during a workday, and the ceiling limit is an exposure that should not be exceeded at any time.

In the United States, OELs have been established by federal agencies, professional organizations, state and local governments, and other entities. Some OELs are legally enforceable limits, while others are recommendations. The U.S. Department of Labor OSHA PELs (29 CFR 1910 [general industry]; 29 CFR 1926 [construction industry]; and 29 CFR 1917 [maritime industry]) are legal limits enforceable in workplaces covered under the Occupational Safety and Health Act of 1970. NIOSH RELs are recommendations based on a critical review of the scientific and technical information available on a given hazard and the adequacy of methods to identify and control the hazard. NIOSH RELs can be found in the *NIOSH Pocket Guide to Chemical Hazards* [NIOSH 2005]. NIOSH also recommends different types of risk management practices (e.g., engineering controls, safe work practices, employee education/ training, personal protective equipment, and exposure and medical monitoring) to minimize the risk of exposure and adverse health effects from these hazards. Other OELs that are commonly used and cited in the United States include the TLVs recommended by ACGIH, a professional organization, and the WEELs recommended by the American Industrial Hygiene Association, another professional organization. The TLVs and WEELs are developed by committee members of these associations from a review of the published, peer-reviewed literature. They are not consensus standards. ACGIH TLVs are considered voluntary exposure guidelines for use by industrial hygienists and others trained in this discipline "to assist in the control of health hazards" [ACGIH 2010]. WEELs have been established for some chemicals "when no other legal or authoritative limits exist" [AIHA 2010].

Outside the United States, OELs have been established by various agencies and organizations and include both legal and recommended limits. The Institut für Arbeitsschutz der Deutschen Gesetzlichen Unfallversicherung (IFA, Institute for Occupational Safety and Health of the German Social Accident

Insurance) maintains a database of international OELs from European Union member states, Canada (Québec), Japan, Switzerland, and the United States. The database, available at http://www.dguv.de/ifa/en/gestis/limit_values/index.jsp, contains international limits for over 1,500 hazardous substances and is updated periodically.

Employers should understand that not all hazardous chemicals have specific OSHA PELs, and for some agents the legally enforceable and recommended limits may not reflect current health-based information. However, an employer is still required by OSHA to protect its employees from hazards even in the absence of a specific OSHA PEL. OSHA requires an employer to furnish employees a place of employment free from recognized hazards that cause or are likely to cause death or serious physical harm [Occupational Safety and Health Act of 1970 (Public Law 91–596, sec. 5(a)(1))]. Thus, NIOSH investigators encourage employers to make use of other OELs when making risk assessments and risk management decisions to best protect the health of their employees. NIOSH investigators also encourage the use of the traditional hierarchy of controls approach to eliminate or minimize identified workplace hazards. This includes, in order of preference, the use of (1) substitution or elimination of the hazardous agent, (2) engineering controls (e.g , local exhaust ventilation, process enclosure, dilution ventilation), (3) administrative controls (e.g., limiting time of exposure, employee training, work practice changes, medical surveillance), and (4) personal protective equipment (e.g., respiratory protection, gloves, eye protection, hearing protection). Control banding, a qualitative risk assessment and risk management tool, is a complementary approach to protecting employee health that focuses resources on exposure controls by describing how a risk needs to be managed. Information on control banding is available at http://www.cdc.gov/niosh/topics/ctrlbanding/. This approach can be applied in situations where OELs have not been established or can be used to supplement the OELs, when available.

Below we provide the OELs and surface contamination limits for the compounds we measured, as well as a discussion of the potential health effects from exposure to these compounds.

Inorganic Acids

Table B1 provides the OELs for the inorganic acids we sampled in the air. The primary health effects from exposure to airborne inorganic acids are acute irritation (from corrosion) to the upper respiratory tract, skin, and eyes [IPCS 2000a,b,c,d, 2001, 2006]. Sulfuric acid can also alter the mucociliary clearance capabilities of the respiratory tract. Long-term exposure to sulfuric acid at concentrations much higher than those measured during this evaluation have been associated with laryngeal cancer [ACGIH 2004]. The OELs are intended to prevent these effects.

Table B1. OELs* (mg/m³) for inorganic acids measured during the December visit

	Hydrofluoric	Hydrochloric	Phosphoric	Hydrobromic	Nitric	Sulfuric
NIOSH REL	2.5 STEL 5	C 7	1 STEL 3	C 10	5 STEL 10	1
OSHA PEL	2.5	C 7	1	10	5	1
ACGIH TLV	C 5	C 7	1 STEL 3	C 6.6	5 STEL 10	0.2[†]

* C = ceiling limits and STEL = short term exposure limits. All other OELs are for 8 to 10 hour TWA concentrations.

[†] Thoracic particle size.

Terpenes

Terpenes are a large class of hydrocarbons found in essential oils and resins of a wide variety of plants, including marijuana. Because terpenes are volatile and aromatic, they can be smelled in the air at very low concentrations. For example, limonene has a reported odor threshold of 10 parts per billion [Leffingwell & Associates 1990]. The terpenes commonly released by marijuana include limonene, alpha-pinene, beta-pinene, beta-myrcene, and beta-caryophyllene [Lai et al. 2008]. Limonene exists in nature as one of two isomers, d-limonene or l-limonene. Of the terpenes released by marijuana, d-limonene is the only one with an OEL. The AIHA WEEL for d-limonene is 170 mg/m³ and is based on liver toxicity observed in rodents [AIHA 1993]. D-limonene can also be irritating to the skin and eyes [IPCS 2005]. Exposures to monoterpenes (like alpha and beta-pinene) ranging from 10 to 214 mg/m³ have been related to acute and chronic respiratory affects to employees in some industries [Eriksson et al. 1996, 1997].

Drugs of Abuse

Methamphetamine, cocaine, oxycodone, and THC (drugs we sampled for in this evaluation) can produce neurological and physiological effects at relatively high doses (milligram levels) [Gable 2004; DEA 2010]. However, the effects from low doses (nanogram levels of indirect exposure) are not well understood. Summarized below are the potential health effects for each of these drugs at its effective dose (for nonmedical purposes), which is the amount of drug that produces the desired response in 50% of users [Gable 2004], and at much lower doses, such as those encountered in occupational settings.

Methamphetamine and Cocaine

Methamphetamine and cocaine are classified as stimulants. The possible health effects from an effective dose of stimulants include increased alertness, excitation, euphoria, increased pulse rate and blood pressure, insomnia, and loss of appetite [DEA 2010]. Studies investigating health effects from lower exposures to these compounds are few. In one notable study, investigators administered surveys to law enforcement personnel to determine symptoms experienced while they investigated clandestine methamphetamine laboratories (after ventilation of the laboratories). More than 70% of the respondents reported headaches, central nervous system symptoms, respiratory symptoms, sore throat, and other symptoms. There was also a positive relationship between the number of laboratories investigated and risk of symptoms [Burgess et al. 1996]. According to an MSDS for cocaine hydrochloride topical solution (Roxane Laboratories Inc., Columbus, Ohio), inhalation of cocaine could cause numbness to the mucous membranes and nasal cavities, nervousness, confusion, and restlessness; eye and skin irritation are also possible [Boehringer Ingelheim Roxane Inc. 2008]. However, this MSDS does not provide an OEL for cocaine.

Because of the large number of clandestine methamphetamine laboratories requiring remediation, several states have adopted feasibility-based surface contamination limits for methamphetamine. Presently, 16 states have adopted surface contamination limits for methamphetamine ranging from 100 ng/100 cm^2 to 500 ng/100 cm^2 [NAMSDL 2008]. These limits are intended to prevent adverse health effects to future inhabitants of buildings that once contained clandestine laboratories. Unlike OELs, these limits consider possible exposures to children, who are more susceptible to the health effects of drugs than adults, as well as economic factors associated with remediation. It is reasonable to assume, then, that maintaining surface contamination levels of methamphetamine below these limits should protect the drug vault employees from experiencing adverse health effects.

Oxycodone

Oxycodone is classified as a narcotic. The possible health effects from an effective dose of narcotics include euphoria, drowsiness, respiratory depression, and nausea [DEA 2010]. No studies evaluating the effects from lower exposures could be found. However, according to the MSDS for OxyContin® tablets (Purdue Pharma L.P., Cranbury, New Jersey), exposure to oxycodone pill dust can cause acute eye and skin irritation, while repeated exposures can lead to skin and respiratory allergies [Purdue Pharma 2010]. Purdue Pharma established an OEL for oxycodone (free base) of 40,000 ng/m^3 to prevent these adverse health effects [Purdue Pharma 2010].

Marijuana

THC is the effective drug in marijuana and is classified as cannabis. The health effects from an effective dose of cannabis include euphoria, relaxed inhibitions, and disorientation [DEA 2010].

References

ACGIH [2004]. Sulfuric acid. In: Documentation of the threshold limit values and biological exposure indices. Cincinnati, OH: American Conference of Governmental Industrial Hygienists.

ACGIH [2010]. Threshold limit values for chemical substances and physical agents and biological exposure indices. Cincinnati, OH: American Conference of Governmental Industrial Hygienists.

AIHA [1993]. Workplace environmental exposure level guide: d-limonene. Fairfax, VA: American Industrial Hygiene Association (AIHA).

AIHA [2010]. Emergency response planning guidelines and workplace environmental exposure levels. Fairfax, VA: American Industrial Hygiene Association (AIHA).

Boehringer Ingelheim Roxane Inc. [2008]. Material safety data sheet for cocaine hydrochloride topical solution. [http://bi-msds.e3solutionsinc.com/COCAINE%20HYDROCHLORIDE%20TOPICAL.pdf]. Date accessed: May 2011.

Burgess JL, Barnhart S, Checkoway H [1996]. Investigating clandestine drug laboratories: adverse medical effects in law enforcement personnel. Am J Ind Med 30(4):488-494.

CFR. Code of Federal Regulations. Washington, DC: U.S. Government Printing Office, Office of the Federal Register.

DEA [2010]. Drug Enforcement Agency (DEA) drug information. [http://www.justice.gov/dea/pubs/abuse/index.htm]. Date accessed: May 2011.

Eriksson KA, Stjernberg NL, Levin JO, Hammarstrom U, Ledin MC [1996]. Terpene exposure and respiratory effects among sawmill workers. Scand J Work Environ Health 22(3):182-190.

Eriksson KA, Levin JO, Sandstrom T, Lindstrom-Espeling K, Linden G, Stjernberg NL [1997]. Terpene exposure and respiratory effects among workers in Swedish joinery shops. Scand J Work Environ Health 23(2):114-120.

Gable RS [2004]. Comparison of acute lethal toxicity of commonly abused psychoactive substances. Addiction 99(6):686-696.

IPCS (WHO/International Programme on Chemical Safety) [2000a]. International Chemical Safety card: hydrogen chloride [http://www.cdc.gov/niosh/ipcsneng/neng0163.html]. Date accessed: May 2011.

IPCS (WHO/International Programme on Chemical Safety) [2000b]. International Chemical Safety card: hydrogen fluoride [http://www.cdc.gov/niosh/ipcsneng/neng0283.html]. Date accessed: May 2011.

IPCS (WHO/International Programme on Chemical Safety) [2000c]. International Chemical Safety card: phosphoric acid [http://www.cdc.gov/niosh/ipcsneng/neng1008.html]. Date accessed: May 2011.

IPCS (WHO/International Programme on Chemical Safety) [2000d]. International Chemical Safety card: sulfuric acid [http://www.cdc.gov/niosh/ipcsneng/neng0362.html]. Date accessed: May 2011.

IPCS (WHO/International Programme on Chemical Safety) [2001]. International Chemical Safety card: hydrobromic acid [http://www.cdc.gov/niosh/ipcsneng/neng0282.html]. Date accessed: May 2011.

IPCS (WHO/International Programme on Chemical Safety) [2005]. International Chemical Safety card: d-limonene [http://www.cdc.gov/niosh/ipcsneng/neng0918.html]. Date accessed: May 2011.

IPCS (WHO/International Programme on Chemical Safety) [2006]. International Chemical Safety card: nitric acid [http://www.cdc.gov/niosh/ipcsneng/neng0183.html]. Date accessed: May 2011.

Lai H, Corbin I, Almirall JR [2008]. Headspace sampling and detection of cocaine, MDMA, and marijuana via volatile markers in the presence of potential interferences by solid phase microextraction-ion mobility spectrometry (SPME-IMS). Anal Bioanal Chem 392(1-2):105–113.

Leffingwell & Associates [1990]. Odor thresholds. [http://www.leffingwell.com/odorthre.htm]. Date accessed: May 2011.

NAMSDL [2008]. State feasibility-based standards. Alexandria, VA: National Alliance for Model State Drug Laws (NAMSDL) [http://www.namsdl.org/documents/RemediationStandardChartFinal.pdf]. Date accessed: May 2011.

NIOSH [2005]. NIOSH pocket guide to chemical hazards. Barsen ME, ed. Cincinnati, OH: U.S. Department of Health and Human Services, Centers for Disease Control and Prevention, National Institute for Occupational Safety and Health (NIOSH) Publication No. 2005-149.

Purdue Pharma [2010]. Material safety data sheet for OxyContin tablets. [http://www.purduepharma.com/MSDSs/OxyContin_binder.pdf]. Date accessed: May 2011.

Acknowledgments and Availability of Report

The Hazard Evaluations and Technical Assistance Branch (HETAB) of the National Institute for Occupational Safety and Health (NIOSH) conducts field investigations of possible health hazards in the workplace. These investigations are conducted under the authority of Section 20(a)(6) of the Occupational Safety and Health Act of 1970, 29 U.S.C. 669(a)(6) which authorizes the Secretary of Health and Human Services, following a written request from any employer or authorized representative of employees, to determine whether any substance normally found in the place of employment has potentially toxic effects in such concentrations as used or found. HETAB also provides, upon request, technical and consultative assistance to federal, state, and local agencies; labor; industry; and other groups or individuals to control occupational health hazards and to prevent related trauma and disease.

The findings and conclusions in this report are those of the authors and do not necessarily represent the views of NIOSH. Mention of any company or product does not constitute endorsement by NIOSH. In addition, citations to websites external to NIOSH do not constitute NIOSH endorsement of the sponsoring organizations or their programs or products. Furthermore, NIOSH is not responsible for the content of these websites. All Web addresses referenced in this document were accessible as of the publication date.

This report was prepared by Kenneth W. Fent, Srinivas Durgam, Christine West, John Gibbins, and Jerome Smith. Medical field assistance was provided by Kristin Musolin. Health communication assistance was provided by Stefanie Evans. Editorial assistance was provided by Ellen Galloway. Desktop publishing was performed by Greg Hartle.

Copies of this report have been sent to employee and management representatives at the police department, the Kentucky Cabinet for Health and Family Services, the Kentucky Labor Cabinet, and the Occupational Safety and Health Administration Region 4 Office. This report is not copyrighted and may be freely reproduced. The report may be viewed and printed at http://www.cdc.gov/niosh/hhe/. Copies may be purchased from the National Technical Information Service at 5825 Port Royal Road, Springfield, Virginia 22161.

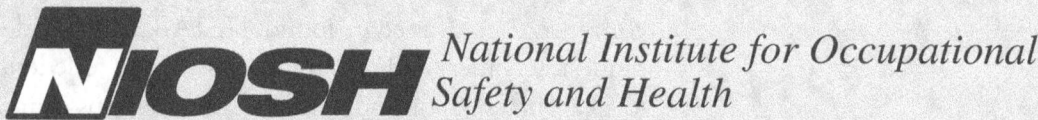

National Institute for Occupational Safety and Health

Delivering on the Nation's promise: Safety and health at work for all people through research and prevention.

To receive NIOSH documents or information about occupational safety and health topics, contact NIOSH at:

1-800-CDC-INFO (1-800-232-4636)

TTY: 1-888-232-6348

E-mail: cdcinfo@cdc.gov

or visit the NIOSH web site at: **www.cdc.gov/niosh.**

For a monthly update on news at NIOSH, subscribe to NIOSH eNews by visiting **www.cdc.gov/niosh/eNews.**

SAFER • HEALTHIER • PEOPLE™